MW01300137

This Journal Belongs To:

____

Made in the USA
Las Vegas, NV
01 February 2023

66653576R00072